The ultimate Sex guide for beginners

Go Beyond Sex

the ultimate guide for beginners to reach great sex and pleasure.

Everything you have to know about sex and everything you must <u>AVOID</u> to get incredible sex and be remembered

Dorian Wilde

Legal & Disclaimer

The information contained in this book and its contents is not designed to replace or take the place of any form of medical or professional advice; and is not meant to replace the need for independent medical, financial, legal or other professional advice or services, as may be required. The content and information in this book have been provided for educational and entertainment purposes only.

The content and information contained in this book has been compiled from sources deemed reliable, and it is accurate to the best of the Author's knowledge, information and belief. However, the Author cannot guarantee its accuracy and validity and cannot be held liable for any errors and/or omissions. Further, changes are periodically made to this book as and when needed. Where appropriate and/or necessary, you must consult a professional (including but not limited to your doctor, attorney, financial advisor or such other professional advisor) before using any of the suggested remedies, techniques, or information in this book.

Upon using the contents and information contained in this book, you agree to hold harmless the Author from and against any damages, costs, and expenses, including any legal fees potentially resulting from the application of any of the information provided by this book. This disclaimer applies to any loss, damages or injury caused by the use and application, whether directly or indirectly, of any advice or information presented, whether for breach of contract, tort, negligence, personal injury, criminal intent, or under any other cause of action.

You agree to accept all risks of using the information presented inside this book.

You agree that by continuing to read this book, where appropriate and/or necessary, you shall consult a professional (including but not limited to your doctor, attorney, or financial advisor or such other advisor as needed) before using any of the suggested remedies, techniques, or information in this book.

Table of Contents

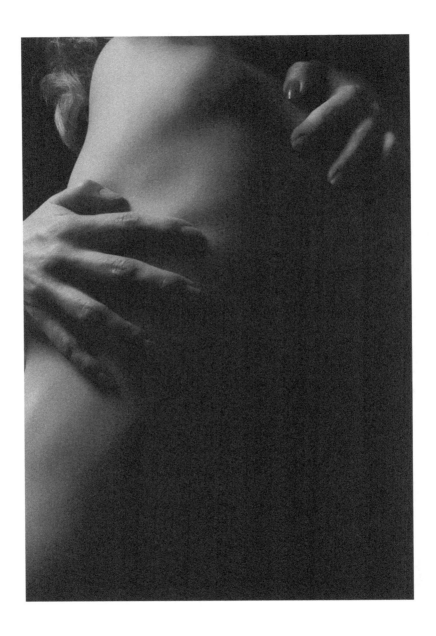

Introduction

Sexual chemistry can be difficult to define, but we will do our best. It is the way our body understands attraction and love without our minds being involved. When you are around someone, and you feel as if a shock runs through your body, it is our body's way of showing us there is chemistry. This occurs because of sexual intuition.

Intuition, in itself, is when we can understand something right away without our conscious playing any sort of role in it. These are our feelings of instinct. Intuition helps us know when we are in danger or in a place of safety. It helps clue us into the intention of the world around us.

The attraction we feel toward someone before we know anything about them is another good way to describe sexual chemistry. It's that magnetism that can simply not be ignored. Sometimes it can be quite overwhelming, while other times, it feels like a simple tug.

Many times, when sexual chemistry is high, it will feel as if you have no control over yourself. Your desire for that individual will overrule your head. It sweeps over people quickly and cannot be denied. It can happen from a look, a touch, or even their voice. You never know what the thing will be that shows you have great sexual chemistry with another person.

Why sex is so important

Longer Life: sex can actually help you live a longer life. Maybe not by twenty years, but can give you a year or two on your life span. The reason is, the more you get into it, the more sex you will have, and sex is exercise. Exercise will help extend your lifespan.

Improved Mood: Along with the increases sex life, you will find that you are in a much better mood. This actually has nothing to do with the sex. It has to do with the emotional connection you will gain with your partner as you two become closer and touch and kiss more.

Restful sleep: This can also help extend your life more. You will sleep better at night due to being fully worn out and satisfied, along with feeling loved and secure in your relationship as you lay next to your partner at night.

Go through this boo and you will need all you need as a beginner.

Chapter 1: Compatibility

Sexual compatibility

This refers to the same beliefs, values, preferences, desires, and expectations related to sex. This can include things like what sex acts you prefer the most, your level of sex drive, the type of sex you wish to have, including any fetishes, and so on. For example, if you have a very high sex drive, meaning that you need and expect to have sex every single day, you will be sexually compatible with someone who also has a high sex drive. If you were in a sexual relationship with someone who had a very low sex drive, this would be incompatible as you would likely become frustrated by their low need for frequent sex. Another example is if you desire a lot of oral sex and you require this in order to become fully aroused during sex, you would be sexually compatible with someone who also enjoys oral sex, especially giving it. If you were with someone who did not feel comfortable with oral sex at all, this would not make for a sexually compatible match.

Discover compatibility

Sexual compatibility, believe it or not, takes time and effort to cultivate. It's not something that happens naturally since sexual expectations and desires differ greatly from each man and woman. Sex is a very personal thing, and even if you have a lot in common with your partner, there will still be differences you might have to work through. Imagine if you had to eat the same food every day for the rest of your life. Same food, same taste, same quantity, same flavor. How long do you think it's going to be before you get tired or bored of it? It's the same thing with sex. If you don't take an active role in keeping the spark alive, it's going to get boring real quick. Yet, many of us still expect everything to fall into place magically when it comes to sex, with little to no effort. When it doesn't, we feel incredibly disappointed, but we don't want to talk about it.

If you believe you've found your perfect match in every way and you don't want to lose that relationship over sexual differences, there is something you could do about it. You and your partner need to work on building your compatibility together and here's how you do it:

- Step 1 – You Must Communicate. You need to get over the reluctance to talk about it and have an open, honest, heart-to-heart discussion with your partner if this is going to work. Communication is not just the key to making this work, it is the foundation on which the rest of your relationship is built on. You and your partner must be willing to share everything right down to your fetishes and kinky desires without holding back if you want to get to the point where a fulfilling sex life is possible. Speak up. Express yourself. Don't be afraid to talk about it if the relationship is worth working on.

- Step 2 – Learning to Compromise. A relationship is hard work, and two people need to be working together as a team on every level for the relationship to work. Even when it comes to sex. The truth of the matter is, no one is ever going to be a 100% perfect match. Some level of disparity will always exist, even in the most perfect couples, and you're going to have to be willing to compromise and sacrifice without resentment on some aspects if you want to be compatible. You're not always going to be in sync all the time, and trying to fulfill each other's desires must be a shared responsibility. The most important thing here is the willingness of both parties to work on the shortcomings.

- Step 3 – Accept Your Incompatibility – As you communicate with your partner, be honest, and accept that you might not be as compatible as you would like. Living in denial only makes it harder. If you don't' acknowledge the problem, it's going to be hard to fix. Healthy relationships have arguments and disagreements, yet you find a way to understand each other and work on your connection. It's the same thing with sexual compatibility. Being a perfect match is a myth you need to let go of. Instead, embrace the problems to find solutions so you can work on becoming more compatible instead of growing further apart.

- Step 4 – Let Go of Unrealistic Expectations – Unrealistic expectations only lead to disappointment. What's worse, you put an unfair and unnecessary burden to live up to your expectations. If you don't communicate what these expectations are, your partner might not even realize they're letting you down. This secret resentment and unhappiness, feeling disappointed by your partner, can quickly lead to the deterioration of a relationship. We're all guilty of having a certain expectation of what we would like our partner to be, but these expectations could also make it difficult for you to find happiness in your relationship if everything isn't exactly how you want it to be. Having expectations and certain standards are fine; it's the unrealistic expectations that you need to start letting go of.

- Step 5 – Listen Without Judgment. You might be reluctant to openly talk about your sexual preferences with your partner because you're worried if it's going to change their perception of you. Maybe they'll even judge you. But you know what? Your partner has those same concerns too. What if their sexual preferences upset you and cause you to leave them? During the communication process, it is important to listen to each other with an open mind. Don't judge, but respect that this is who your partner is, and this is what they like and vice versa. Everyone is entitled to their preferences, and no one should have to be made to feel ashamed of them if these preferences are healthy sexual desires.

What not to do when building compatibility

As you work on building your sexual compatibility with your partner, these are the common mistakes that you want to avoid:

Don't Tell Them What They Want to Hear

It cannot be emphasized enough how important honesty is here. Don't tell your partner what you think they want to hear just to keep them happy. You need to be honest right from the start of your relationship of it's never going to work in the long run.

Don't Try Too Hard

We all want to impress our partners in bed, but not to the point that we compromise our sexual happiness by trying too hard to please theirs. Both partners should be equally happy and satisfied, and there should be an equal amount of giving and receiving that goes on.

Don't Be Reluctant to Try

Now that you've talked about it, ideally, the next step is going to be that you try out some of your partner's preferences to satisfy them and vice versa. Avoid being too reluctant to try it out, be willing to give it a go at least once before you decide whether this is something you enjoy or not. As the old saying goes, don't knock it until you've tried it.

Chapter 2: How to talk before sex

Communication is the key to a fulfilling and pleasurable sex life. Knowing what you and your partner like and dislike allows you to focus on the things you enjoy and leave the things you don't behind. Knowing this will help to greatly reduce your anxiety surrounding performance or being able to please tour partner adequately. With so many options for ways to pleasure each other, you don't want to waste time on the things that don't make you scream out in pleasure, and communication is the way!

Talking Before Sex

What you both like and don't like:

In terms of sex acts, this could be anything like oral sex, fingering, anal, and other butt stuff or anything that she enjoys, no matter how big or small. These could be things she has tried before, wants to try in the future, has never tried before, or that she knows she does not want to try. Keep this question very open-ended to get the maximum amount of information possible.

What you both need and like during foreplay specifically:

This could include the length of time she needs, what acts she likes done to her, and what she likes to do to you during foreplay if she likes kissing to be included or not and what it takes to get her into the mood and wet enough for penetration.

What you both like and don't like specifically that you do or have done:

These are things specifically related to the two of you having sex with each other. The other questions in this list are open to including anything in her past and anything she has not yet tried. Try not to take it too personally if she tells you there is something she does not enjoy as much as you thought she did. This conversation is all about growth and learning.

What, if anything makes you both orgasms almost instantly?

Maybe something she does for herself during masturbation, or something she knows will set her off instantly in the best way. This could be something you do for her or something she likes to do for herself.

What both of your favorite positions are:

Her favorite sex positions, both for penetrative sex and for sex not involving penetration. What she likes about them would also be beneficial for you to know.

Any kinks or fetishes you both may have:

Both that she has experience with and that she is just discovering. If she is unsure, ask her if she is open to exploring new kinks with you. Maybe you both will find new things that you really enjoy.

Anything you both have wanted to do sexually specifically with you:

Maybe you have never done a 69 together, but she enjoys this position, or maybe she saw something in a porn video that she would like to try. Maybe there is something that she has wanted to experiment with, and she is wondering if you would be open to it.

Anything you both have been fantasizing about trying:

Maybe a role-play or a specific location, maybe a fantasy that she is embarrassed to talk about. This question is last on the list because hopefully, at this point, the conversation is flowing a little easier, and she will be more comfortable answering this question by now. Make her feel comfortable and let her know anything she discloses to you will remain between you and her.

While these questions are extremely personal, you will have to make each other feel comfortable being open about these topics. This will require a lot of vulnerability on both of your parts, so show your partner that you are listening intently and assure them that you are doing so without judgment. If they seem very hesitant to open up about these things- and they might be, depending on the age of your relationship and each of your levels of openness with sex in general, you can ask them if they would rather you answer the questions first, and they can answer them afterward. This may make them feel less like they are on the spot (especially if you were the one that brought it up) and more comfortable with the conversation as a mutual exchange.

When it comes to sex, communication is key to ensure everyone has a happy ending.

Chapter 3: Orgasm

What does she want?

The first thing that happens physically when a man or woman becomes aroused or any kind of stimulation begins is that the heart rate increases. This leads to an increase in blood flow and immediate delivery of blood into the genitals and the surrounding areas as blood vessels dilate. This is where the differences begin between the genders.

Women not only have an increase in blood flow to their genitalia but also to their breasts which may cause them to swell and slightly increase in size. The breasts, along with the vagina, are flushed with fluids that cause them to feel firm and even as if they are pulsing. From here, women can continue the stimulation or action that has helped get them to this point until they reach their peak of orgasm. Female orgasms are more difficult to bring about to completion than male orgasms, but they can also last up to a minute longer than male orgasms (making them well worth it in most women's opinions).

What does he want?

For males, once the blood flow and heart rate have increased, their genitals will grow in length and become firm (similar to the female reaction). As the sexual activity continues (be it foreplay or intercourse), the genital muscles go through a series of contractions, tensing and releasing as reproductive fluids are pushed into the urethra to be ejected once the male reaches his climax and peaks. Men have less difficulty inspiring and achieving release, but their orgasms tend to be shorter (an issue that can easily be overcome through building sexual endurance).

Best sex position for male orgasm

Cowgirl

Make him rests on his back, mount yourself over him with every leg on either side of his middle. Instead of bouncing all over, you can concentrate more on moving your crotch to and fro, scouring your clitoris on his open and paunch district. You can likewise pound your pelvis around and around while Kneeling. It causes you spread your legs more extensive. Keep your hand laid on his chest, cause him to sit in a semi-inclined position where his back is leaned against the casing of the bed.

Being on top gives the lady unlimited authority with respect to the speed, pace, profundity and movements. Men additionally last longer as this position is easy for them, and they simply can sit and appreciate, snacking at your areolas, kissing your neck and lips, squeezing your bosoms and crushing your body.

Best sex position for Female orgasm

Doggy Style

This position involves the female resting on her hands and knees while the male (or partner doing the penetrating) positions themselves behind her, standing or on their knees depending on the difference in height and which is more comfortable and effective. From there, the penetration begins and continues to reach further as the intercourse continues. The reason this position is so successful for achieving female orgasm is that the angle at which the penetration happens gives the partner almost direct access to the G-Spot and that access is uninterrupted by tangling legs or other complications that can arise from different positions.

Chapter 4: Erection and Ejaculation

Tips for stronger erections

Patience

The journey will not be all rainbows and sunshine but with commitment, persistence, and patience, you will pull it off. There is no cure for PE. You will need to combine medications and exercises. The exercises will take time to see results. However, if you stick to your carefully planned routine, then you can enjoy an improved sex life too. You will make more than a few errors, but if you keep at getting it right, you will succeed.

Visualization

Having an optimistic outlook plays a substantial part in the outcome and satisfaction you develop when overcoming any obstacle. By erasing the negative aura and effect of the shame associated with premature ejaculation, you will discover sex to be more pleasing and perform longer than expected. Irrespective of how you are feeling: take a moment, remove from your mind the word impossible, and instead focus your mind and energy on what is possible.

Masturbation Before Sex

If masturbation is useful for premature ejaculation, does it mean you should masturbate before sex? This is a technique that men with premature ejaculation have exhausted thinking you should masturbate now to "get it off your mind," so you can perform longer during actual sex.

Quite sadly, it is not as easy as masturbating before sex to slow down ejaculation. It is a temporary fix, not a logical long-term approach. In my observation, older men find it hard to retain an erection once they have masturbated, while young men find it easy to retain an erection during actual sex.

Consider this before you start

The relaxation of your body helps you to fight anxiety and focus on the pleasure of sensations. Furthermore, it helps you reduce your sexual arousal. If you do the exercise separately from the previous exercises, start with 2 to 3 minutes belly breathing. Sit comfortably on your chair/couch/bed. Close your eyes and relax. Start breathing from your belly, counting to 3 as you inhale and again to 3 as you exhale.

Observe your toes, feet, calves, and thighs. As you observe each part one by one, feel the tension leaving from your body. It would help, if during the exhalation you imagined that a burden leaves from these body parts and goes down to the floor. Feel your two legs completed relaxed. Breathe calmly and deeply. Feel the air as it goes in and out of your body.

Healthy Habits for stronger and longer erection

Get to the gym

Cardio is going to be your new favorite word if you want to keep your penis healthy and strong enough to maintain its rock-hard erection. Aerobic workouts encourage blood flow in the body. There's a lot of benefits that come with exercise. It keeps you strong. It keeps you in shape. It builds the nitric oxide in your body, the one you need to maintain your strong erections. Just scale back on the cycling, those tight shorts don't do your penis and testicles any favors either.

Watch your time on your bike

If you're an avid cycler, you might want to watch how much you spend on your bike, as some research suggests erectile dysfunction could be caused by the pressure that is put on your blood vessels and pelvic area. Consider investing in a better bike seat that doesn't place too much pressure on your perineum.

Get Enough Sleep at Night

Never underestimate the importance of what getting enough sleep can do for your overall health and sex life. Inadequate sleep has been linked to an increase in experiencing erectile dysfunction. A lack of sleep is also likely to lead to plaque developing in your arteries, affecting your blood circulation. When the circulation is affected, maintaining an erection becomes increasingly more challenging. Get the recommended seven to eight hours of sleep at night and watch what a difference it makes to your sex life.

Tone Down the Stress

It's a difficult request, but for the sake of your erections, you need to try. Either minimize or manage the stress as best you can, so it doesn't affect you as much as it otherwise would. Research links erectile dysfunction to psychological conditions like anxiety and stress. Of course, stress could lead to other conditions, too, including high blood pressure, higher cholesterol levels, heart disease, and obesity, none of which are good for your erections.

Scale Back on The Nicotine

Or better yet, don't use it at all. Cigarettes, vaporizers, cigars, none of that is doing your erections or your body any favors. Nicotine damages your blood vessels, which makes it difficult to maintain an erection. The sooner you quit cold turkey, the happier your sex life will be.

Pour That Cup of Coffee

Cigarettes and alcohol may be bad for your penis health, but coffee is not. As it turns out, the University of Texas' Health Science Center found that men who consumed two to three cups of coffee in a day were less likely to experience erectile dysfunction. Scale back on the sugar and try to keep it to black coffee, so you're not overdoing it with the sugar intake.

Cock Rings

Sex toys come in handy once again, and this time, it' the cock ring to the rescue to help you maintain your erections for longer. Slipping the ring around your penis helps to keep the blood in your shaft, which is exactly where you want it to be. Cock rings are also helpful for preventing venous leakage, a condition where the blood has no trouble flowing to the penis, but it has trouble staying there. Venous leakage is a form of erectile dysfunction too. With the cock ring putting a stop to that, your blood stays where you want it and keeps your erections stronger for longer. Try adjustable, solid, stretchy, or vibrating rings, depending on what you and your partner prefer.

Food for greater erection

- Avocado
- Garlic
- Watermelons
- Pumpkin Seeds

- Oysters

- Almonds

- Figs

- Bananas

How to delay ejaculation

The strategies mentioned in this book will point you in the right direction when it comes to improving your sexual stamina, but there are still a few more strategies that can be used to prolong your orgasm while you are practicing and getting used to these exercises.

Your first choice is to use a condom during every sexual encounter you have. For apparent reasons, this is safer and it also numbs your penis and prolongs sex. They are easily available and will help to prolong the length of your sexual relations.

Secondly, select a style and master it.

Reflecting on the masturbation strategies we discussed previously, if the slow technique helped you last longer, then practice that in your bedroom and do the same for the withdrawal technique. Also, just a while before reaching orgasm, pull out and reduce the pace of your thrusts.

Keep in mind to control your breathing and deploy the strategies that were mentioned in the breathing chapter of this book.

If your lover is interested, normalize the atmosphere by engaging in a light conversation. This distraction technique can help to eliminate the pressure to ejaculate and it distracts your mind from arousal.

Another strategy to delay your premature ejaculation is to practice thrust control when you are close to ejaculation and you can do this by becoming attentive to the period when you are almost there, decrease the pace of your thrusts or completely penetrate your partner without thrusting to decrease your excitement levels. Remaining in there, without action, is not something so absurd. You can consider it as another form that you have to enjoy and feel your partner, try to capture its temperature, its internal dimensions, try to listen to its micro convulsions. Personally I think this is a technique that gives a lot of intimacy to the couple. Yes, because many times, as mentioned above, we take too much care to do and not to hear. You also allow her to notice and enjoy your presence. Remember, there's no hurry.

How soon is too soon?

Premature ejaculation is among the most common complaints that men have sexually. An estimated 1 out of every 3 men would agree that they have experienced this problem at some stage throughout their sexually active years. It isn't a cause for alarm unless it happens too frequently. How soon is considered too soon and falls into the premature ejaculation category? Well, a medical professional might diagnose you with the condition if you frequently ejaculate within a minute or two after penetration, can't delay your ejaculation nearly or all the time, and you feel distressed enough about it to avoid getting sexually intimate with your partner.

Symptoms to watch out and how to avoid them

Symptoms

The most obvious symptom would be your inability to delay your ejaculation. However, the symptoms of premature ejaculation are not confined to intercourse alone. It could happen in all sorts of sexual situations, even masturbation, when you're going at it alone. Coming too early falls into the premature ejaculation category if:

The exact cause of premature ejaculation is not known since each man is different. Biological and psychological factors have a role to play if you find yourself struggling to control your ejaculation. Psychological factors include:

- Dealing with stress and anxiety, including performance anxiety. You're worried about losing your erection, and that worry combined with the trauma of having it happen in the past is going to affect your ability to control yourself.

- Depression

- Relationship troubles

Then there are physical problems that could be the culprit, including:

- The sensitivity of the penis

- Lower threshold for ejaculation

- Erectile dysfunction

- High blood pressure

- Hormonal imbalance

- Alcohol

- Erectile dysfunction

- Side effects from other medications you might be taking

- An unbalance in your brain's chemical balance

- It is inherited

- Infection or inflammation of your urethra or prostate

Psychological triggers of early ejaculation could come down to:

- What your early sexual experiences were like

- Any sexual abuse you might have experienced in the past

- A lack of confidence and poor body image

- Feeling guilty that you're dealing with this

It's time to see your doctor if, again, it happens more frequently than it should. It is normal for men to feel embarrassed talking about this since troubles in the bedroom make a lot of men feel like they are "less of a man" somehow, but don't let that stop you from going to a doctor if you think you might need some extra help. Premature ejaculations are perfectly normal, and more importantly, treatable. Talking to your doctor about it could help relieve some of the pressure you may have been feeling about this.

The obvious risk factors of this condition would be the stress that it causes in your relationship. If the stress is severe enough, it could lead to the breakdown of the relationship entirely. Then there are the fertility issues that this condition might pose. Ejaculating prematurely will make it difficult for you to have a baby if the ejaculation doesn't happen intravaginally.

How to avoid them

When you see your doctor about this condition and explain what you're dealing with, your doctor is going to talk to you about the physical symptoms before performing an examination. Some blood tests might be suggested, depending on your results if your doctor feels there is a need to find out what the underlying causes of your condition may be. Tests are not always necessary.

The treatment you might need to overcome this condition would depend on two things. The first is whether you're dealing with primary or secondary ejaculation, and the second is what your relationship status us. A combination of treatments often works best, depending on how you respond to them. Possible treatments to have you overcome premature ejaculation might include some of the following:

- Seeing a sex therapist for help

- Seeing a couple's therapist so you can work through your issues with your partner

- Medication

- Treatment for any co-existing or underlying medical problem like erectile dysfunction.

Other techniques to last longer and give longer pleasure

Communication with your partner is key to help you work through the next few techniques. Despite the way it makes you feel, continually remind yourself that dealing with early ejaculation is not the end of the world. There is a solution for every problem, that's one of the greatest benefits to living in the modern world we do today. There are several natural techniques you can work on by yourself or with your partner to help bring this situation under control before medication is brought in as a last resort. These techniques include:

The Start and Stop

Allow your partner to stimulate your penis in this technique long enough until you feel like you are about to ejaculate. When you feel close, let your partner know it's time to stop the stimulation. Wait for about 30-seconds or so, and then begin the stimulation again, repeating the process. This exercise, when done for a period of time can you improve your control over your ejaculation.

The Squeeze

Another common technique used is by withdrawing your penis or putting a stop to foreplay before your orgasm hits. Stop, and then squeeze the end of the penis where the head and the shaft are joined. Keep applying pressure on the squeeze until you feel your urge to ejaculate pass. Resume your regular sexual activities.

Kegels

These exercises could be of some help to you here. By strengthening your pelvic muscles, you give yourself the upper hand. You are the one in control, and if you can learn to control your urine stream midway, you can learn to control your ejaculation the strong your pelvic muscles become.

Chapter 5: Anxiety

Why are you anxious?

Anxiety in men can be a consequence of a mental issue or physical.

Physical causes: mental or physical ailments can bring problems in a man's sexual capacity. These ailments bring vascular (vein) and heart malady, hormonal uneven characters, neurological issue, continuous illnesses like liver or kidney failure, abuse of alcohol and misuse of medication. Sexual want and capacity can be influenced by symptoms of specific drugs such as energizing drugs.

Mental causes: These include relationship or conjugal issues, wretchedness, worry about sexual execution, business related nervousness and pressure, a past sexual injury, and sentiments of blame.

How to overcome Anxiety

Communication

During sex is an important time to check in with your partner to see how they are feeling, what they are liking, and what they want more of. While you are having sex, it is easiest to communicate using dirty talk so that you don't ruin the mood by coming off too serious or too concerned. In order to properly communicate while also playing into the mood of the moment, you can do so in a sexy way, using sexy language. You should tell each other what you like by saying, "oh yes, I like that" or "I like when you touch me like that" This lets the person know to do more of the same because this is what will get you to orgasm. By being aware of these things and being able to talk about them at the moment, it will help with your confidence in the bedroom and reduce your insecurities.

Environment

Your choice of environment can make a big difference when it comes to whether or not you can reach orgasm. If you tend to be someone who has trouble reaching orgasm for whatever reason, these details of the environment, the location, and the time will be important for your experience. They will determine whether or not you will be able to get concentrated enough to orgasm. We will discuss several factors that contribute to whether or not your environment is conducive to your pleasure and your orgasm. The reason why the environment, time, and location are of such importance is that being comfortable with all of these factors will allow you to focus on yourself, your pleasure, and your orgasm without distraction.

Exercise

If your insecurity stems from an inability to reach orgasm, as orgasms are not easily achieved in times of stress and anxiety, this technique can help you to improve your likelihood of anxiety.

Cardiovascular exercise has been shown to increase blood flow, which in turn increases your positive feelings during sex as well as the sensations your partner will feel on his penis when he slides it into your engorged vagina. Improving your aerobic capacity makes it so that blood will have an easier time flowing to the genitals, as your body becomes more efficient at dispersing it. This means positive things for your orgasm as well as your partner's! In terms of sex drive, doing weight training has been shown to increase your sex drive, which is another factor that will positively affect your ability to orgasm. Another one of the countless benefits of exercise on your sex life is that it will make you feel more confident and positive about your body. This, in turn, will make you feel more confident in the bedroom, which will improve your mood, reduce your stress and anxiety, and make it so that you are more likely to reach orgasm.

Sex position to overcome anxiety Foreplay to easy it up

The Deep One

In this, the woman makes herself as open to penetration as possible. This she does by lying flat on her back and getting into a comfortable position.

Once she is in place and ready, she can rock gently backwards until she can pick her legs up and hold them high in the air. This should leave her lover with no misgivings about what he needs to do next. He has full access and considerable encourage to take her then and then and fill her yoni with his full and ready lingam.

Chapter 6: Lubricant

Lubrification during sex Types and use

Using lube alone is not enough. You need to consider the type of lube if you want to create some magic between the sheets. Some lubes can cause allergic reactions or irritations if you're not careful, and there is nothing worse than feeling like that burning sensation on your penis or vagina.

Water-Based

These are the most versatile out of all the lubes and safe for all sexual activities. They are even safe to use on sex toys, making water-based lubes are the most popular choice. They're inexpensive, easily available, doesn't stain and is safe to ingest in small amounts during sex (read the list of ingredients first though). Don't worry if you're using diaphragms or latex condoms. They're safe to be used on these products too. Water-based lubes are the popular choice among women because it feels like natural vaginal lubrication. Plus, they are incredibly easy to wash off once you're done, leaving your skin clean and residue-free.

Oil-Based

For a long-lasting, smooth, and silky experience, oil-based lubricants are a good choice to consider. Since they are thicker and creamier, they last longer during sex too. If you're masturbating, oil-based lubricants can be a great choice, but be cautious with these since not all oil-based lubes are safe to use when there are latex contraceptives involved. Oil-based lubes can be combined with water-based lubes during sex.

Silicone-Based

These last a very long time and a great if you're planning to get frisky in the water. They are also safe to use on latex condoms, but the downside is that it's not the best idea to use them on silicone sex toys since they will damage the surface area of the toys.

Petroleum-Based

These you want to stay well away from if you can since they are difficult to wash off and could cause some irritation by altering the vagina's pH levels. This could potentially lead to yeast infection, and plus, they destroy any latex-based products that you might be thinking about using them on. Not a great idea.

What not to do

Don't Forget the Ingredients

Never buy or use lube without reading the ingredients. Some lubes might contain ingredients you or your partner may be allergic to, and the last thing you want is a trip to the hospital because of a bad reaction, either one of you had. Some lube ingredients could cause UTI, so always err on the side of caution by reading, reading, reading.

Don't Experiment If You're Not Sure

If you want to play it safe, its best to stick to water-based and silicone-based lubes just to be safe.

Don't Forget a Test Patch

When purchasing any new lube, always do a test run on your hands first. It's better to let your hands bear the brunt of what might happen and not the sensitive tissues of your genitals where the damage incurred could be much worse. Even if you're buying from the same company but a different variety, always do a test run beforehand.

Chapter 7: The Magic World of Oral Sex

Oral sex for male

Get It Really Wet

Make sure the penis gets really wet; otherwise it won't be an enjoyable session. Obviously, saliva would be the main thing used as a lubricant. However, if you're partial to a little bit of flavor, then edible oils would be the perfect accompaniment for the oral pleasure. You'll find that there are literally dozens of possible flavors out on the market today so you won't have any problems finding one that works best for your needs.

Rhythm and Pace

The whole point of a blow job is to simulate penile-vaginal intercourse which means that you don't have to go fast and furious from the get go. Instead, use different speeds, pace, and depth so that your lover doesn't know what to expect next. It's perfectly OK to go slow first and then hit a fast pace and then go slow again. There's no specific speed or count just follow your mood as well as pay attention to the signals of your partner.

Hardness May Vary

According to experts, it's not necessary for an erection to stay hard all through the fellatio. In fact, hardness may peak and ebb during the process so don't worry too much if your man gets a little softer during the oral game.

Oral sex for Female

Get Her Comfortable

Receiving oral sex for men is easy not so for women. The position isn't exactly comfortable which is why it's important if you give her time to really get into position. Possibly the most comfortable position for oral sex would be lying down with pillows piled high under her pelvis. This tilts up the vagina and allows for a large opening, thereby giving you lots of room to work. In this position, guys also get lots of control and comfort so that they can play as much as they want.

Lick and Suck

Biting or nipping may be good for some guys receiving oral pleasure, but it's always a negative for the girls. Feel free to suck and lick as much as you want, but never let her feel the teeth because it will definitely bring her out of the moment.

Play with the Lips

The lips or labia is wonderfully sensitive, especially when it comes to light pressure. Using the edge of your tongue on this body part will definitely send shiver down her spine, especially if you follow up with a good and long hard suck.

Locate the Clitoris

Know where the clitoris is located and have fun with it. Note though that the clitoris shouldn't receive all your attention. Remember that in this position, you have access to both the clitoris and the U-Spot which is that sensitive plump flesh just a few centimes below the clitoris.

Listen and Learn

If you're not getting encouragement – either verbal or physical – you're probably not doing it right. Most women would moan or do something that tells you you're hitting the right spots. There are also instances when she'll grab the guy's hair and direct the movement of the lips and mouth, silently telling him where to go and which part to focus on. The tilting and shifting of the pelvis is also indicative of this particular need. Make sure to pay attention to these changes so you'll be able to fully give her the orgasm she wants or needs.

Not Just the Mouth

Note that oral sex isn't completely oral. In the same way the women use their fingers when giving a blow job, men can also use their fingers during oral sex. In fact, it's usually a better idea since their fingers can enter and stretch the vagina in such a way that men can stimulate two important points all at once: the clitoris and the A-Spot. If men are particularly good, they can also hit the U-Spot and the K-Spot at the same time.

Best oral sex tips

It mustn't be just oral sex

You can start off with oral sex and finish up with penetration. You can stop off with mild foreplay, penetrate, and finish off with oral sex. It doesn't have to be oral sex alone. Also, this doesn't mean it can't be orals sex alone.

You and your partner can have an orgasm from oral sex alone.

Don't stop after they cum

Even after your partner has had an orgasm, keep going for a short while.

Watch porn

Watch porn together or let your partner alone watch porn while your head is buried in between their heads.

This can be used to set the mood at the beginning or increase sexual tension while oral sex is still ongoing.

Talk dirty

Before you go fully into oral sex, it is good to set the mood and create a more intense sexual tension by talking dirty to your partner. Tell them all the things you are going to do to them, whisper to them how hot their body is and how turned on you are by them. You can say something like, 'Oh baby, I can't wait to get a taste of your sweet juice, you'll eat you so hard, you will forget your name. I'm so hard I can shoot a truckload of cum in your face,' It doesn't have to be these words exactly, but do you get my point?

Best oral sex position

The 69

The 69 is a good oral sex position for reciprocity. This is to say, the couple gives themselves oral at the same time, mutually. This can be overwhelming as each couple is being pleasured while trying to focus and perform oral sex on the other partner.

It is easy to get into and stress-free. The 69 position is better done on the bed or a soft surface. This is for the lovers to be comfortable.

In this position, the couple lies on their sides with the man's head on the woman's pelvis and the woman's head on his too. The woman can take the man's penis in her mouth and do as she likes with it. The man can also do the same. However, if the height difference of the couple is too apparent it may be challenging to get the best out of oral sex in this position.

The Corkscrew

In corkscrew oral sex position, the man stands, and the woman gets in front of him and lowers herself to his penis. She could kneel on her calf, so she doesn't get weary of supporting herself entirely on her knees.

In the corkscrew position, the penis is right before her, and she takes it from there. This position is one of the easiest positions for her to perform oral sex on the penis. She can hold it in her hand and position it in any way she likes. She can also tilt her head to any position of her choice.

The man can hold her head and mildly guide her as she thrusts her head back and forth.

All Hail the Queen

In this position, the man lies on his back, and the vagina sits on his face. The woman who is on top can easily adjust until she is at the angle the oral sex is most pleasurable.

To get in this position, the man lies on his back. The woman gets on her knees on top of his head by straddling him. Her knees are on either side of his head. This way, her vagina is directly above his mouth. She can lower herself till her vagina is closest to his mouth without suffocating him.

As the man person the oral sex, he can grab her waist to hold her in place.

The Spiderman

The Spiderman sex position is another thrilling position that pleasure the partner on top. The man lies on his back with his head on the edge of the bed but not over it. The woman stands right in front of him and bends down till her hands are on the bed by his side. She should be close enough that when she bends, her vagina is just over his head. She can also spread her legs apart so he can have a good assess to her wet vagina.

He can then begin to perform oral sex on the vagina she has presented to him. This position is comfortable and straightforward for both partners.

What you should never do

Ignoring Her Other Hot Spots

It's easy to get lost in the focus of your attention, but your lover's body is covered with erogenous zones just dying for some equal attention. So, don't ignore your lover's nipples, bum, or back of the knees, just to name a few of the favorite parts within arm's reach.

Not Easing Off the Clitoris

Every girl is different when it comes to how much her clitoris can handle stimulation, and this varies. Sometimes, she may want it hard and direct. Other times, she may need you to ease off on her crown jewel, providing indirect or no stimulation. This can be in the very same oral sex session. So be sure to check in with her and to tune into verbal and nonverbal cues that she may need more or less of whatever you're doing.

You're Not Present

You had a tough day at work; you're feeling gassy from gorging yourself at dinner; you're wondering when you'll find the time tomorrow to pick up your dry cleaning …. There could be a million reasons why you're not into oral. But even if you're not into the moment, pretend that you are. Make sure that your hands are busy, exaggerate your head movements a tad, make some noise … pretty soon you may even start to believe your own performance and really get into everything you're doing.

Chapter 8: Anal Sex

For many people, the thought of anal sex is extremely intimidating. This simply does not need to be the case. Anal sex can be truly enjoyable for both men and women. We have stated several times that you need to be willing to experiment. This is one of those areas that you should really give a try before you completely say no to it. Communication is extremely important and there is definitely information that you need to be aware of before entering into this type of sexual situation.

How to enjoy it better

Use your tongue

It is not only the penis and vagina that oral sex can be performed on. When oral sex is performed on the anus and the area around it, it is known as rimming. In this technique, use your tongue and stimulate the amuse like you would a vagina if you have tried that. Tease the cheeks with the tip of your tongue and the area around the anus. Then work your way to the anus and its erogenous zones. Also, you can try to push the tip of your tongue in and out of the anus.

Lubricate

During anal sex, use tube generously, apply a little more, and then some more. This cannot be said enough. Because the anus does not get wet naturally, you need to get it wet artificially to aid the movement of the penis and to reduce friction. If the anus is not well lubricated, it can easily lead to skin tear and pain.

There are different kinds (not just brands) of lube, so it is important to find which works for you and your partner. However, silicone-based lube is more recommended than other forms of lube. It is very silky and smooth and can last throughout the sex without drying up. It is also compatible with latex condom, so there is little risk of the condom ripping.

However, when choosing a lube, it is important to pay attention to the brands and the ingredients used in its production. Some contain ingredients that can damage the anal tissues.

In cases when you want to have unplanned anal sex, and there is no lube insight, you can use saliva. This is not the best option and can easily dry out, but it is better than nothing. Never attempt to have anal sex with no lube.

Where to start

Anal sex is the form of sexual intercourse that involves the anal area. It includes the sexual stimulation of the anus and rectum and areas around it. It is basically the penetration of the anus, finger, sex toy, or the desired object into the anus and rectum and thrusting to induce sexual pleasure. Anal sex, however, isn't limited to the insertion and thrusting of a penis or a toy into the anus. It also includes the use of the tongue and mouth to stimulate the anus and anal area for sexual pleasure.

During anal sex, the anus produces a tightness around the penis that can result in intense sexual pleasure. In comparison to the vagina that is more elastic, the anus clings around the penis more firmly and creates a tight sensation. Anal sex is not just pleasurable for the giving partner. There are many nerve endings in the anus, making it erogenous; and sensitive to sexual pleasure. So, the receiving partner is not left out of the fun.

Anal sex is a form of sex that is adventurous but even more pleasurable for many than other kinds of sex. Its animalistic nature is a source of thrill for many. Also, it can be performed on anyone who has an ass hole, which is virtually male and female! So anal sex can be practiced by gay, straight, bisexual, transgender people, and people will all kinds of sexual orientation.

Position for starting

Back Entry

In this position, the couple has more skin to skin contact, and as a result, it aids intimacy. The receiving partner lies on their belly and spreads their legs apart. The giving partner, usually the man, gets on top, facing the same direction as the receiving partner. He props himself on by placing his hands by the sides of his partner. He enters his partner.

The rear-entry position supports closeness, body contact, and intimacy. Its downside, however, is that it can be uncomfortable for the receiving partner if the giving partner on top is overweight or has a big stomach. The weight will put pressure on the back of the receiving partner, and this can make sex not so enjoyable. To curb this, the giving partner has to be careful not to lean down so much on his partner.

Advance position for better anal sex

Tea spooning

Tea spooning is an intimate anal sex position that aids body contact and connection. This position lets the couple explore their bodies with their hands, and the penis makes its way inward and outward in the anus.

To get into this position, the receiving partner gets on her knees without slouching. She kneels upright. The man does the same thing she has; gets on his knees behind her uprightly. He enters her in this position.

The tea spooning position lets the couple wrap their hands around themselves. The woman can reach back and hold the man closer to her. This fosters intimacy and, at the same time, helps her maintain her balance. The man can also caress her breasts, fondle with her vagina and generally let his hands wander around her body.

The advantage of this position is that it is easy to get into, and as mentioned earlier, it aids intimacy between the couple. However, as the couple is both on their knees, they do not have a strong balance, so the pace of thrusting in this position is more slow than fast. This is a downside for couples who want to go all-in and rough. However, a remedy to this is couples who engage in this position do so in front of a wall. This way, the receiving partner can push back against the man. This would act as a support, and the man can be rougher.

Missionary

I bet you didn't know that a missionary position was possible during anal sex. Well, it is. In the missionary anal sex position, the couple can make eye contact, wrap their hands around themselves and even kiss.

To get in this position, the woman lies on her back and spreads her legs apart. The man gets on top of her, propping himself up with his hands. The woman's legs are on either side of him, so she can curl them around him if she chooses. The man penetrates her anus in this position just as he would during virginal sex. She can place a pillow under her buttocks to move her hips closer to him.

The missionary anal sex position is easy to get into and fosters intimacy. They can make eye contact, the woman can wrap her hands around him, and he can bend and kiss her.

Lotus

This is a variant of the lap dance position, but unlike the lap dance position, the couple can make eye contact and are more intimate.

The man sits on a chair, sofa, couch or bed and crosses his legs. The receiving partner gets on his laps and wraps her legs around his hips. He penetrates her in this position.

The lotus position is not very easy to get into and requires some flexibility from the couple. Also, if the stomach of the couple is big, performing anal sex in this position will be uncomfortable. Another downside of this position is that the movement of the lovers will be quite limited. To solve this, the woman can bed her knees and place her feet on the surface behind him. This will give her more control and help her move her hips more easily.

The advantage of the lotus anal sex position is that it is very intimate. The couple can share deep eye contact and even kiss. Also, the woman can wrap her hands around the neck of the man, while he wraps his own hands around her waist or hips.

Chapter 9: Toys

Vibrators and sex toys

Aside from a penis, a tongue, or fingers, a vibrator can be a woman's best friend. If you're a woman that doesn't have a vibrator (you poor, deprived thing!), you might want to consider getting one. Not only is it a great masturbation tool and a fine stress reliever, but it's also a wonderful way to share a sexual experience with your partner. Vibrators come in a variety of different shapes, sizes, styles, etc. You can get the old school, white plastic model, or you can go for the ultra-realistic looking dildo in the shape and size of your favorite male porn star.

How to get the best out of it

Some people view sex toys as something that is for those who have wild kinks or those who cannot perform without assistance of some sort. In reality, though, sex toys are designed to increase and enhance pleasure for anyone. By using sex toys, you do not have to engage in anything wild or anything that you are uncomfortable with. You are also not admitting that you have a sexual problem by using a sex toy.

One of the ways in which sex toys can improve your sex life is that they allow you to focus on one area of the body while the sex toy takes care of pleasure in another. For example, a sex toy that is designed to pleasure a woman's clitoris will do so while you can focus on her nipples or her vagina.

Finding the right toy

In order to choose the right sex toy for yourself, there are a couple of questions that you would need to answer first.

- Is this toy to be used alone during masturbation?

- Is it to be used with a partner?

- Is it to be used with multiple partners?

- Is it to be used for all of the above or two of the above?

- Do you want it to have a vibrating function?

- An insertion function?

- Will you use it anally?

- Vaginally?

- Both?

- Do you want it to be customizable (depending on your mood or the partner you are with)?

Once you establish this, you will be able to narrow down your search. Answering all of these questions will help you to determine which type of sex toy is right for you (and your partner).

Sex position and sex toys

Once you've got your first four sex toys ready, it's time to combine this with some sex positions and begin exploring just how much pleasure the introduction of something new can bring. Of course, you can start getting a little more adventurous later once both partners are comfortable with the idea of using these toys in the bedroom. Until then, these positions will serve as a good first step to test the waters:

The Missionary with Vibrator

Time to get back to basics once more as you slowly familiarize each other with the use of these sex toys. The woman will be lying down on her back on the bed, relaxed and ready. The man starts off slow and gentle, locating her clitoris with his fingers. Turn the vibrator on a low buzz, slowly bring it between her legs and place it so that it lightly touches her clitoris. The man then watches her facial expressions change as he tries varying amounts of pressure and speed settings of the vibrator. Occasionally take her by surprise by slipping a finger inside her vagina and find her G-spot while the vibrator is still going. Listen to her moans of desire for your cues to help her reach intense levels of pleasure. Adjust the speed when you're ready, increasing the speed as the woman gets wetter and wetter.

Doggy Style with The Strap-On

The Doggy position, when combined with a strap-on creates a mecca of pleasure. This time, however, it is the man who is going to be in the Doggy position while the woman wears the strap on and do what you normally would do in this position. Be careful when playing with the man's anus, and don't forget to use lots of lube for this one.

Seated Sex Position with the Vibrating Cock Ring

With the Cock Ring positioned at the base of the man's penis, vibrating and ready, the man sits in a chair while the woman sits on his lap, facing him with her legs around his waist and behind you. Have her stand up slightly, so she is hovering before she lowers herself onto the vibrating penis. Work together to move her body up and down on your penis. She can rotate her hips slightly backward, and the vibrating ring should stimulate her clitoris. The vibration of the ring will give her intense pleasure, and this position is ideal for a great male orgasm and a great female orgasm too.

Chapter 10: Masturbation

Man's secret pleasure point

Male masturbation is described as the act of a man pleasuring himself by either touching or stimulating his penis, nipples, testicles, and other erogenous zones in his body. These self-pleasuring techniques usually carry on to the point of ejaculation or orgasm, and it is done purely to satisfy his sexual pleasure. This can be done either solo or when you're in private or as part of the foreplay leading up to sex with their partner, although most of the time, masturbation typically happens when the man is alone. As a man, masturbation can help you deal with anxieties, understand your sexual preferences, your body, improve your endurance during sex and generally keeps you happy.

Woman's secret pleasure point

Masturbation can be just as life-changing for a woman's sex life as it can be for a man. Many women struggle with body issues and poor self-image, but masturbation is a way of overcoming that and learning to love your body as it is. When you know how to pleasure yourself, it makes it easier to guide your partner about what they need to go to take your orgasms to the next level. Self-love is important for a woman because it can deeply affect your intimacy with your partner when you're not comfortable in your own skin. If you haven't spent a lot of time pleasuring yourself before this, it's never too late to start.

First, get to know your body better by holding a mirror between your legs to see what your partner sees when they are touching you or giving you oral sex. Take a good look at what you look like down there. This is you. This is your body. Now, start to feel around a little bit, massaging your vulva and locating your clitoris. Play around the area and observe the way your body responds to the touch. Some areas will feel oh so good while others will feel very, VERY good. You want to keep the sensation going on the "very good" areas.

Hand tricks to give extreme pleasure

Masturbation is often thought of as a solo act, but it could be surprisingly pleasurable to do this with your partner. Masturbation is an intimate thing and sharing this moment with someone you care about can bring you closer together as a couple. Mutual masturbation can be an incredible moment shared between you and your partner. For the man, watching his partner masturbate is probably high on his sexual wish list. It may not be as high on the list for the woman, but you may be surprised at how arousing it could be. As a bonus, you may each learn something new about your partner's arousal process. Some women may never even have seen a man ejaculate in real life other than is watched in porn films. Men, ejaculating in front of your partner is a very intimate act, and surprisingly enough, many women find it arousing not only physically but mentally and emotionally.

Face-to-Face

This position can be pulled off in a few ways, depending on how you and your partner like to do it. Begin by lying down on your side, facing your partner, and gazing into their eyes. The closer you are, the greater the intimacy and intensity of the moment. Touch yourself the way you would if you were masturbating alone and watch your partner's face start to change as they pleasure themselves too. It's a great time to throw in some dirty talk here. Keep this going until you both climaxes, perhaps even try attempting to orgasm at the same time.

Don't Ask

Instead of asking for sex, show your partner that you're in the mood instead. This tip works best for women, and without saying a word, position yourself provocatively comfortably and make sure he's got a good view. Place two fingers in an inverted V straddling your clitoris. This hand position is good for encouraging your orgasm. Throw yourself into your masturbation session with abandon and watch his face start to change as continues watching you pleasure yourself.

Stimulating His Testicles

This secret is key to giving your man some of the best orgasms of his life. This secret is in the testicles and knowing how to use them as a secret weapon of pleasure. Cup your partner's testicles gently and begin stroking them softly. Hold them and very lightly pull them towards you (be gentle here because his testicles will be sensitive to your touch). To double the pleasure, give him fellatio while you do this, it's going to drive him crazy as the stimulation of both his penis and his balls at the same time will make it hard for him not to finish right then and there. The warmth and moisture of your mouth around his penis, along with his testicles being gently rubbed will lead straight to orgasmic bliss.

Chapter 11: Spice it up with dirty talks

What to say and when

That sometimes difficult, but always necessary sex conversation is what we are going, to begin with. This conversation can be difficult to work up to, especially if you have not had many conversations like this outside of dirty talk in the bedroom. What I'm talking about is an adult conversation where you ask them what they want, what they need, and what they like and dislike. This conversation is one that should happen in every relationship when you first begin a sexual relationship and should be revisited over and over again throughout the course of your relationship, but it is never too late to have this conversation for the first time.

Communication Outside The Bedroom

The best way to communicate outside the bedroom is to have a conversation at a time when you are both unaroused, and your feelings won't be clouded by sexual frustration. If, after talking about this, you are both so horny that you go and jump on each other in the bedroom, that's fine, but begin this conversation in a different time and place so that it can be a serious dialogue about both of your needs.

Communication During Sex

During sex is an important time to check in with your partner to see how she is feeling, what she is liking, and what she wants more of. This is also a time where you can tell her what you like and what you want more of. While you are having sex, it is easiest to communicate using dirty talk so that you don't ruin the mood by coming off too serious or too concerned. In order to properly communicate while also playing into the mood of the moment, you can do so in a sexy way, using sexy language. You should tell each other what you like by saying, "oh yes, I like that" or "I like when you touch me like that" This lets the person know to do more of the same because this is what will get you to orgasm. If your girl seems like she is really enjoying what you are doing, don't change it up, keep doing the same. With a woman, if you find that thing she likes- don't give it up! It may be hard for you both to find the spot she likes and the way she likes it, so if she is getting hot and bothered by the way you are touching her, keep it up. If she does not usually communicate this, you can ask her in whatever way she is comfortable while you have your sex talk we discussed earlier. You can ask her to let you know when she likes the way you are touching her and let her know that this will help you to give her great orgasms.

Communication After Sex

Next time you have sensual pillow talk, ask them what their favorite part was. Ask her what she liked and what you did that was different than before. You can open up this dialogue by telling her how sexy you thought she was or how you liked it when she did a certain thing to your penis. After sex is a good time for this because it is fresh in your minds and you can revisit it together while you both still remember exactly what you did to each other.

Chapter 12: Make it more sensual with Erotic Massages

Tools and technique for better massage

Erotic Massage

This type of massage is focused around the genitals and the erogenous zones in general. The aim of this massage is not necessary to give the person an orgasm, but it is very likely. The goal of this type of massage is to make your partner feel sexual pleasure and relaxation, but it is different from sex in that it involves the focus being solely on one individual.

Female Erotic Massage- The Yoni Massage

A Yoni Massage is a vaginal massage that is intended to open up the woman to her sexuality, her pleasure, and her sexual desires. As a partner, you can perform this type of massage for your woman to unlock her repressed sexual energy and help her to get in touch with it.

This can be done in a variety of ways, but the position we are going to discuss is a Yoni Massage. Begin by setting the ambiance, either in the bathroom with a bathtub, or in the bedroom. Set up some candles, some flowers, or anything that will make the surroundings relaxing and calm. Begin by having her breathe deeply and focus on her body and its sensations. You can get into the bed with her for added intimacy. Begin by slowly and gently massaging around her entire vulva and her clitoral area. The key to this type of massage is to do everything very slowly. Begin to massage her clitoris slowly and not with the intention of making her come. When ready, and with lots of waterproof lube, slide one finger inside of her vagina and gently begin massaging the upper wall. Here is where her G-spot is located. Encourage her to express and release any sounds she naturally makes. Move your finger in a circular motion slowly and with your other hand, massage her pelvic area and clitoris. This connects the inner with the outer. Continue to do this and let the experience unfold with no end goal in mind. If she reaches orgasm, she can do so, but if she doesn't, she can just enjoy the pleasures that she is getting from your massage. As discussed earlier, this massage is intended to reconnect a woman with her pleasure and allow her to focus on herself and her body. After this massage, she will feel more in touch with her body, and if penetrative sex ensues, both of you will feel even more pleasure and intensity of orgasms because of how engorged and activated her vagina and clitoris will be.

After doing this practice for some time either with you or on her own, she will be more in tune with her body all of the time and not just when doing this practice.

This will lead to stronger orgasms overall and hotter sex for both of you.

Male Erotic Massage- The Prostate Massage

A sort of erotic massage that you can try giving to a male partner is the prostate massage. As you know now, the prostate is a small gland located inside a man's body between the base of his penis and his anus. It is accessed through the anus. This type of massage is similar to anal play, but it is not the same, as the goals are different, and so is the technique. The reason why it is better to give a man an erotic message here instead of on his penis is because he will be able to last much longer without reaching orgasm.

Performing this type of massage requires lots of lube for maximum comfortability. Once your fingers are well-lubricated, you can slide a finger or two inside of the man's anus very slowly. As we discussed previously, you will have to go slow so as not to shock the anus into closing tightly. You will need to work your way in gradually. Once in, you will be able to find the prostate by feeling around on the upper (front) wall of the rectum for a small lump that is rough in texture a few inches deep. Once you have found it, you can begin to gently massage it. You can move your fingers in circles and apply light pressure to it. This massage has the potential to feel quite pleasurable for the man. Communicate while the massage is occurring in order to give him the most pleasure possible.

You can perform this type of massage in a number of different positions. The man could be lying down while you straddle his legs, he could be on his hands and knees while you sit or kneel behind him, he could lie across your lap while you sit on a bed, or you could do any position that is comfortable for you.

This massage does not need to lead to orgasm; at least that is not the goal. If it happens, that is fine. However, the aim of this massage is just to provide a relaxing and pleasurable experience for him.

Chapter 13: Tantric sex

The word 'tantric' comes from the Indian tantra which means a written text. These texts were known as threads or fundamentals because their subject matter invariably concerned important issues such as sex, religion or the attainment of enlightenment. A tantra was the written equivalent to a mantra, a spoken chant or prayer which could bring about a union with God if used correctly and repeatedly. Likewise a yantra was a drawing or painting, usually geometric that could achieve a similar result if studied hard enough or meditated upon.

How to further improve your sex life

Spanking

Spanking is a becoming an increasingly popular activity for fun loving couples. As with everything else in this book, its two-way street and one which both of you can enjoy giving and receiving? You may want to incorporate it into your role play, with one of you playing the principal to the naughty school girl/boy. Lights! Cameras! Action! You may even need costumes.

Spice Up Your Sex Life

There are many ways to spice up your sex life, and as you learned there is a lot beyond the bedroom that can be done to enhance it as well. This chapter will explore some ideas of what you can do to make your sex life even better outside of the bedroom.

Do Fun Things Together

Doing fun things together allows you to increase your dopamine levels together as well. When you have fun together, it increases your closeness with one another and can enhance the joy you experience with each other. It adds a unique sense of intimacy to your relationship that cannot be added by sexual experiences.

Kiss More Often

Many couples, especially those who have been together a while tend to kiss less often. Kissing is a highly romantic and passionate act and should be done regularly. Think about it, at the beginning of the relationship you likely kissed your partner a lot more frequently than you do now that you are more comfortable together. You want to start doing it more often.

Describe Your Sexual Fantasies

Many times, sex is just about the act and couples don't really speak a lot about sex outside of the bedroom. A great way to spark up a flame and add passion to your sex life is to talk about each other's fantasies and interests. This gives you an opportunity to get to know each other's sexual preferences more intimately which means that you can gain maximum enjoyment out of sex. It allows you to have a better idea of what your partner likes and what they don't like, and how you can make sexual experiences more enjoyable for them.

Chapter 14: Sex lifestyle

Improving sex life with food and exercise

Working hard at the gym is no longer for aesthetic and health purposes alone. Sure, looking toned and fit can enhance your level of attraction, but regular exercise can improve your flexibility, sexual techniques, stamina, and endurance in the bedroom. Some of the advanced moves covered in the previous chapters require a great deal of strength and flexibility, and regular training with the following exercises will eventually lead to better sex as you get stronger and fitter over time:

Squats (Men and Women)

Some sexual positions can demand a lot from you, and the stronger your legs are, the more fun you and your partner will have in the bedroom. Squats target the hamstrings, quads, glutes, and the pelvic muscles too.

Lifting Weights (Men)

Men do quite a bit of the heavy lifting in most of the sexual positions, and strengthening your muscles with regular training will prep you for any position you might be keen on being adventurous with. Weight lifting for men encourages the release of testosterone, a precursor for sex drive in men. Studies have even linked weight lifting to higher testosterone levels. Sit-ups, push-ups, and crunches are great for building and strengthening your chest, shoulders, and abs. Men need a strong upper body to increase stamina levels and keep your partner moaning for longer.

Kegels (Men and Women)

Men and women can both benefit from Kegels to enhance endurance and tone the muscle group known as the pubococcygeus (PC). If you have ever tried to stop your urine flow mid-stream and succeeded, that's the PC muscles at work. Strengthening your pelvic floor muscles can help delay ejaculation when your muscles are strong enough to contract before an orgasm. Kegels can be practiced at any time, and a good place to begin would be in the toilet. The next time you're answering the call of nature, try stopping your urine flow mid-stream several times.

Yoga (Men and Women)

Strengthen your body from every angle and prepare to take on some of the more advanced sexual maneuvers by regularly using yoga for exercise. Yoga enhances both strength and flexibility, and learning to control your breath and flow of energy means your stamina is given a boost.

Swimming (Men and Women)

A Harvard study was done on 160 females, and male swimmers discovered that regular swimmers in their

60s had better sex lives that were comparable or better to swimmers in their 40s. Swimming enhances endurance, and if you can swim for long distances, you can go on and on in the bedroom for a long time too.

The Bridge Pose (Men)

Keeping the pelvic muscles strong is the key to thrusting harder and for longer periods. Bridges are also great for strengthening the hamstrings and the glute muscles.

Frog Jumpers (Men and Women)

This move is explosive and very tiring because it requires maximum energy exertion in a short space of time. It's a great strength-building move that will help with a lot of the advanced sexual positions you've been curious to try.

Planks

This move looks simple, but it is an overall body workout that will enhance stability and strength. All you need is your own body weight as you work on your balance, upper body, and core strength, which will make those challenging positions easier to handle when balance is not an issue.

Eating for better sex

Avocados

A healthy sex drive requires a dose of B6 vitamins and folic acid, both of which can be found in avocados. B6 vitamins help to stabilize your hormones, while folic acid gives your energy levels a boost.

Apples

Rich in quercetin and antioxidants, apples help to promote blood circulation.

Peaches

Take your sperm count numbers up by including more peaches into your diet. The high level of vitamin C in these fruits helps minimize infertility issues.

Dark Chocolate

There's always a good reason to indulge in some chocolate. It may not boost your libido, but dark chocolate can trigger the release of endorphins and serotonin, which significantly improve your mood. Feeling happier means sex is better.

Garlic

Eating garlic before or while you're on the date is one the oldest dating advice around. But it turns out this pungent herb could be the extra flavor you need in the bedroom. Garlic is a natural blood thinner, and its anticoagulant properties will keep the blood flowing to your privates.

Walnuts

Help enhance sperm quality, including boosting its movement and vitality. If you're looking for a food that's going to kick your fertility up a notch, start snacking on some walnuts.

Almonds

The arginine in these nuts helps to relax your blood vessels, which then improves circulation. They are especially beneficial for men who want to maintain a healthy erection for longer.

Raspberries and Strawberries

Loaded with zinc, these berries are great for both men and women. When women have higher zinc levels in their bodies, it's easier to get in the mood. In men, zinc helps to control the level of testosterone in the body.

Watermelon

Men who chow down on their fair share of watermelon have healthier erections and a higher libido. The citrulline contained in watermelons releases amino acids and arginine into your system, too, the latter being responsible for vascular health.

Coffee

Spike up your sex drive with this stimulant and take your arousal to greater heights.

Oysters

Possibly the most famous name associated with aphrodisiac foods.

Saffron

Oysters are not the only aphrodisiac, saffron is too, although it doesn't get quite the same level of fame that oysters do. Looking to boost energy and stamina in the bedroom? Give saffron a try.

Wholegrains, Fiber, Seafood, Legumes

The American Heart Association recommends these food groups keep your circulatory system in tip-top condition. A good working system is essential for better sexual health in both men and women.

Salmon

Packed with omega-3 fatty acids that keep your circulatory system running and blood flow moving, salmon, tuna, and halibut are the fishy friends you need to enhance your sexual experience.

Red Wine

Another classic dating staple from the scenes you see on TV is a glass of red wine. Research done by the Journal of Sexual Medicine states that red wine is beneficial for women, and it helps put them in the mood for sex. Two glasses of red wine could increase lubrication and sexual desire in women, probably because of the quercetin found in this substance. However, the researchers did note that other alcoholic beverages didn't give quite the same result.

Proven supplements for better sex

There are various supplements that have been proven to make sex better. Some of those supplements are:

- Zinc
- L-arginine
- Ginseng
- Vitamin D3
- Sandalwood Essential Oil
- Vitamin B12
- Ashwagandha
- Collagen Protein

Move to last longer and get better sex

Performance anxiety is the main reason for premature orgasm. Studies demonstrate that men who approach sex with less certainty are generally less mindful of their excitement levels and are likewise seldom in control of their ejaculatory process. Thusly, they seldom keep going long, and they fail to fulfill their partners. The thoughtful framework that is produced under Tantra theory ordinarily concentrates on giving a man all-encompassing wellbeing and peace and consequently expanding a man's certainty regarding the matters of the bedroom. The very viable reflective methodology is likewise successful in managing both physical and enthusiastic apprehensions of a man and thus permitting the man to have sex with his whole being.

Any sex specialist will let you know that an incredible sexual execution more often than not requires a considerable measure of persistence since it is the moderate development of sexual force that makes for the best climaxes. Tantric sex tips normally concentrate on helping couples to control their reactions to sexual excitement while putting a considerable measure of accentuation on taking as much time as required when having intercourse. The focus is generally on closeness and not moment fulfillment of a physical sexual inclination. By underlining the association of the heart, brain, body and soul, these standards bring about more extraordinary and more enduring climaxes.

Make love during period

There are some benefits that come from having sex on your period. One of these benefits is that having sex while on your period can actually offer relief from the pain of period cramps. Period cramps can be very painful, and anything that makes them feel better is a welcome suggestion, especially when it feels as good as sex will. This result is because of the orgasm. The chemicals that are released in the brain make you feel happy and also have pain relief functions. The other reason is that an orgasm makes the uterus contract and then release. The release part of this will likely make a woman feel better than she did before in terms of cramps.

Another benefit of having an orgasm during your period is that it leads to the uterus contracting, which actually pushes the blood and uterus contents out faster, leading to a shorter period length. This also means that there is ample natural lubrication and that lubricant is not necessary during period sex.

Sex during pregnancy

Brought down circulatory strain

In spite of the fact that your pulse might be bring down directly subsequent to engaging in sexual relations, it's just brief so the cure isn't sex constantly,

Faulkner said. Since hypertension can be not kidding for both you and your infant, it's critical to work with your specialist on approaches to anticipate or control your pulse.

Enhanced confidence

With every one of the progressions that occur amid pregnancy, it can feel that your body is never again your own. However engaging in sexual relations can help re-establish your body certainty and positive emotions about yourself.

Stress decrease

In spite of the fact that pregnancy is typically a cheerful time, it's ordinary to stress over things like work, funds and how your life will change after your infant is conceived. Oxytocin, the affection hormone that your body discharges when you have a climax, can refute some of that pressure and furthermore enable you to rest better.

Enhanced associations

Having successive sex now will help reinforce the private relationship and bond you have with your accomplice and build up a sound propensity for what's to come.

It's vital to interface with your accomplice now while you have time since you will require that association once the child is conceived

Planning for work

In case you're full-term or past your due date, having intercourse won't place you in the process of childbirth, yet it can enable your body to get ready since semen contains prostaglandins which can help mature the cervix.

Condoms and other anti-conceptional Health and safety

Safe sex is clearly significant, which for some may incorporate security. For men, have condoms all set before you get occupied so you're solid and steady. What's more, realize the best possible approach to put a condom on a partner's penis. I generally suggest obtaining enormous size condoms since there is a tiny distinction among ordinary and huge sizes.

Conclusion

Do you want to have more and more sexual pleasure for you and your woman, and wondering about lasting longer in bed with her? Have you tried to know the reason why your X-girl friends left you? Not all the time but sometimes it's because of your weak sexual performance.

According to a researcher, it is proved that about 40% of breakups we based on this problem. And most of the times your partners declare their decisions without saying or asking anything. So, don't you ever ignore the problem because it's a matter of your life and just because of this small issue do not let your loving partners go away from you.

Because it's tough to find a partner who fulfills every desire of yours and nothing could be able to replace this type of loss.

Start with the easy sex positions as you work your way up through intermediate ones and eventually the advanced positions. A significant first step in making sexual stimulation should be through seduction, which expresses your swish to make sexual advances. Keep in mind that it can be hard to circumvent a partner who is unwilling to try out new sex positions or explore additional sex variants. Therefore, you should approach them with respect and love and persuade them of the need for trying out something different, and it may be a step to indulge in an ecstasy of sexual stimulation and orgasm.

If you feel that you have witnessed some changes, you should keep on implementing these points and continue to repeat it. Just in case, you feel that there is not a lot of change; we want you to go through the lessons once again in the book. Make sure that you do not simply read it, implement each of them.

All the best!

CPSIA information can be obtained
at www.ICGtesting.com
Printed in the USA
LVHW081521110520
655369LV00032B/2315